Paleo Diet for Beginners

Clean Recipes for Losing Weight Fast!

Erin Bloomfield

© 2017

©Copyright 2017 by Erin Bloomfield – All rights reserved.

Table of Contents

Introduction

Due to intensive commercialization and marketing strategies, people are convinced into thinking that fast food and processed food are convenient, practical, affordable, and safe. This may be true in some levels, but these foods are also the reason why many people are suffering from autoimmune diseases, Diabetes, cardiovascular diseases, and cancer.

People are now more aware of the bad effects of processed food. This is why **clean eating** is gaining more popularity than ever. The term and concept of **clean eating** have been around for years but modern day living makes it harder to achieve. That is why **Paleo Diet** was discovered. Among all known diets, Paleo is the healthiest as it mimics our ancestral diet, which is based on **lean meat, fruits, and vegetables.**

This book will help you understand:

- What is healthy eating
- What is Paleo Diet and how is it different from others; and
- Healthy kitchen fundamentals

You will also find delicious and healthy **recipes** in this **cookbook,** including:

- Paleo Soups
- Paleo Salads
- Paleo Lunches

- Paleo Snacks
- Paleo Desserts
- Paleo Dinners

Going clean and healthy eating is easier than you think. This book will help you achieve your health goals with Paleo Diet.

Chapter 1 – What Is Clean Eating

Clean eating is not a new concept. This term has been around for years, although it is gaining popularity nowadays. As the term implies, clean or healthy eating means you choose to eat, natural food rather than commercially processed products that contain all sorts of chemicals and preservatives.

Clean or healthy **eating** is more than just **diet** and it does not have a specific time frame. It is a lifestyle and is meant for a lifetime. Due to modernization and commercialization of foods, it is harder to look for naturally grown foods that are free from pesticides and other harmful chemicals. When you cannot find fresh, whole, organic foods, choose the one that is less processed. Always check the labels. If the product contains ingredients that you haven't heard of or the list of ingredients is more than three, you should have a closer look take it.

The best place to find fresh, organic fruits and vegetables is in the farmer's market. But if you live in a city, where it's impossible for you to get hold of fresh fruits and vegetables, you can opt for the fresh produce section in your local grocery store. They do offer fresh fruits and vegetables, but most of the time, they are not organic. To reduce the chemicals in your fruits and vegetables, soak them for 10 minutes in a basin full of tap water and 2 spoons of white vinegar. You will notice dirt settling at the bottom of the basin. Rinse your fruits and vegetables in running water with a dash of white vinegar or lemon juice and allow them to dry.

You can also take advantage of locally produced fruits and vegetables. They are easier to find and are cheaper when in season. You can also make use of dried fruits or nuts and even packed vegetables. Just make sure they are non-GMO, preservative free and have no additives.

When cooking, use herbs and spices to flavor your food. Do not use artificial flavorings and seasonings such as MSG, bullions and seasoning mixes. You can use salt but sparingly. Too much salt can also cause health risks and diseases. Refined **sugar is a big no-no**. If you need to sweeten your food, use **Stevia** instead. You can also make use of raw honey or maple syrup. Refined sugars are known to cause blood sugar spikes which can lead to Type II Diabetes. They also contain empty calories which make you feel hungry faster and let you crave for more sugar. This is why a lot of children in the United States are obese. Because they are exposed to food and beverages that contain refined sugars.

Clean eating is not just for you. It can be a **diet** for your entire family. As you get healthier, so does your family. **Clean eating** also promotes cautiousness and awareness. Before you buy your food, you cautiously check the labels first and make sure they do not have preservatives and additives. It also makes you aware of the origin of your food. Farmers take time to plant and take care of your food. So it is only right that you prepare enough food that you can finish.

While it is pleasing to the eye to see such bountiful food on your table, putting them to waste afterwards is not a good practice. **Clean eating** does not mean you cannot eat what you want; you just have to eat what is right. Remember, everything in excess leads to something bad. Cook in proportions. If you need to save time, cook in batches and store them in containers that are enough to be consumed per meal. You are not only being socially responsible, you also save more time and money while staying **healthy**.

Chapter 2 – What Is Paleo Diet and How Is It Different From Others

Modern diseases are mostly due to unhealthy lifestyle and unclean eating habits. Americans splurge on foods rich in calorie such as burgers, mayonnaise, hotdogs, salami, and other processed foods. These foods are high in transfat, salt, and cholesterol, which can lead to cardiovascular diseases, diabetes, high blood pressure, and obesity.

These modern diseases can be prevented if you switch to a healthier lifestyle and **diet**. Paleo Diet is about getting **healthy** by choosing your foods and changing your lifestyle. It is based on the **Paleolithic diet** wherein our ancestors ate fruits, vegetables, and meat (yes meat!) that are fresh, non-processed and chemical free.

It is believed that the human body is biologically adapted to whole foods such as plants, meat, and seafood. At the onset of agriculture some 10, 000 years ago, modern foods such as sugar, wheat, seed, and vegetable oils were introduced. It is during this time when many diseases started to spread. These diseases include Type 2 Diabetes, cardiovascular diseases, excessive obesity, and autoimmune diseases. That is not a coincidence. This is why nutritionists and health experts believe that the "caveman diet" is the best approach to eating.

What sets Paleo apart from the other diets is that it's easy and simple to follow. Here's why:

- There is no need to count your **calorie intake.**
- You don't need to **deprive** yourself of your **favorite foods.**
- You are in **control of what you eat.**

- You can enjoy great **tasting food** without hurting your pocket.
- The foods that you consume are **filling and nutritious**; there is no way you can overeat.

Your Guide to Paleo

Food manufacturing companies alter the natural composition of food and add additives to make them more palatable and saleable. These commercial foods are all over the market because they are cheap and can be consumed instantly. This makes it more difficult to look for foods that meet the Paleo Diet criteria.

To make it simple, follow this basic scheme:

You can eat:

Fish
Seafood
Grass-fed or Pasteur-raised Meats
Fresh Fruits
Fresh Vegetables
Eggs
Nuts
Seeds
Healthy Oils

Avoid eating:
Cereals
Legumes (peanuts included)
Refined Sugar
Dairy
Processed Foods
Potatoes
Refined Vegetable Oils
Hydrogenated Oils

You don't even have to worry about the proportions of the food you eat. As long as you have fruit, vegetables, and real meat on your plate, you have nothing to worry about. If you are trying to lose weight, minimize your fruit and nut intake and add up on your vegetables and healthy protein.

Fats have been considered bad for the longest time. But that is not entirely true. According to epidemiological and scientific studies, **omega-3 fatty acids** and monounsaturated fats significantly reduce the risk of cognitive decline, heart diseases, cancer, and obesity. Food companies vilified and demonized fats so that they can sell everything non-fat and low-fat processed foods.

Despite what these big companies have been telling us, not all fats are bad for your health. It is not the amount of fat that you consume; rather, it is the type of fat that you eat that matters. Unsaturated fats and Omeg-3 fatty acids help with your mental health, fight fatigue, help manage your mood and help control your weight. **Trans fats**, on the other hand, are the bad fats. They cause an array of diseases, **clog the arteries**, and causes **unhealthy weight gain**.

You can get your good fats and oils from these sources:

Avocados
Natural peanut butter (contains only peanut and a reasonable amount of salt)
Olives
Almonds
Macadamia Nuts
Hazelnut
Cashew
Pecan
Walnuts
Sunflower Seeds

Sesame Seeds
Flaxseeds
Pumpkin Seeds
Salmon
Tuna
Mackerel
Sardines
Trout
Herring
Soymilk (Non-GMO)
Tofu (Non- GMO)

These healthy fats are not meant to be exposed in high heat as it can alter their natural composition and damage them. They are recommended to be used in cold salads or low-heat cooking only. When nuts or oils start to smell, taste rank, bitter or go rancid, discard them right away and refrain from using.

The secret to Paleo is to **keep it simple**. You can always prepare complicated recipes during your free time. But, if you are in a hurry and have not much time to spare, just whip up some fresh veggies and pre-made salad dressing, take some fruits and nuts and you are good to go. It's good practice to prepare some sauces and dressings in advance and keep them in the fridge to save time.

You can also take advantage of modern conveniences while on Paleo. Incorporating modern technologies with your Paleo **diet** can make it much easier for you.

Chapter 3 – Healthy Kitchen Fundamentals

A **healthy** kitchen does not need any special equipment or tools. It's the same set up as with your old kitchen, albeit the foods that you store are healthier and natural. Paleo Diet consists mostly of fruits, vegetables, lean meat, and seafood. For you to save time, money and effort, it would be best to store some of your food and buy them in bulk.

For starters, clean up your kitchen and let go of anything that has preservatives, artificial seasonings, refined sugars, and unhealthy oils such as refined and hydrogenated oils. Stock up on dried herbs and spices. If you store them properly, they can last longer. Keep them in tightly sealed containers and away from direct sunlight. This ensures their freshness and potency.

It is also wise to have small containers that are enough to accommodate your meals. Resealable bag containers and glass containers are great, especially for sliced fruits and vegetables. If you are preparing your meals ahead of time, you have to mark your containers. Write down the date of preparation and the name of the recipe on the container, so you can easily distinguish which one to cook or consume for the day. Remember the rule: first in, first out.

A blender or food processor is a great addition to your healthy kitchen. Since you will be gorging on fruits and vegetables, it is nice to be able to enjoy them in different ways. Since fruits and vegetables are best eaten raw, a smoothie is a great way to be healthy. You can precut your fruits and vegetables ahead of time and store them in the freezer. When you need a smoothie, just pour the precut ingredients in your blender and you have a healthy drink that is enough to provide you your daily dose of vitamins and minerals.

It is wise to prepare your food for a week during the weekends so it won't affect your daily tasks. It is important that you list all the ingredients you need for your chosen dishes for the week. Keep a small notebook or journal that you can use to write down the things you need to buy. This will help you keep things organized and won't miss anything from the grocery store.

Printing your recipes for the week and hanging them in front of your refrigerator will help you remember what to cook. Label them according to what day you plan to do them. Since your ingredients are already prepared and stored in the refrigerator, all you have to do is bring them out and cook them accordingly. It is important for you to keep your ingredients as fresh as possible. Make sure to set your refrigerator accordingly or everything will go to waste.

If your schedule is really tight and you don't have time to cook your food, a slow cooker can help you tremendously. Before you sleep at night, place all the ingredients in your slow cooker and set in your desired setting. Leave it on and your food is ready by the time you wake up. All you need to do is prepare the food you will bring to your office for your lunch and snack.

Make sure to use BPA-free containers for storing your food. If possible, use glass containers as they are more ideal for storing food. You are trying to go healthy, so make sure your kitchen tools and containers are chemical-free as they can seep into your food.

Chapter 4 – Paleo Breakfasts

Breakfast needs to be fulfilling and healthy as it will fuel your body for the rest of the day. These Paleo breakfast **recipes** are easy to prepare and the ingredients are available in most groceries.

Beef Mexicana

Ingredients:

2	Egg
1	Red Onion
1	Green Bell Pepper
1	Red Bell Pepper
½ cup	Ground Lean Beef
¼ cup	Salsa
1 pinch	Salt
1 pinch	Ground Pepper
2 tablespoons	Olive Oil, divided

Directions:

1. Heat your frying pan over medium heat. Add olive oil and sauté onions. Season with pepper.
2. Mix in ground beef and add salt. Cook until brown.
3. Turn off heat but leave the pan on the stove. Add salsa and mix thoroughly.
4. Transfer in a serving plate.
5. In the same pan, add the remaining olive oil and heat.
6. Fry the egg to your desired doneness. Place on top of ground beef. This dish is best served warm.

Raspberry Chia Pudding

Ingredients:

6	Dates, seeds removed and cut into cubes
1 can (13.5oz)	Coconut Milk
1 tablespoon	Vanilla Extract
1 – 1 ½ cups	Fresh Raspberries (you can use packed raspberries as alternative)
8 tablespoons	Chia Seeds

Directions:

1. In the blender, process coconut milk, vanilla extract and dates. Start from low going to high until smooth.
2. Add raspberries and blend on low for about 1 to 2 minutes. Do not over blend.
3. Mix in the chia seeds until mixture becomes thicker.
4. Transfer in glass containers and refrigerate overnight for a thicker pudding.
5. Serve with fresh fruits on top.
6. It stays fresh in the refrigerator for 3 days. Make sure container is properly covered.

Banana Pancake

Ingredients:

2 large	Overripe Bananas, peeled and mashed
2 tablespoons	Raw honey/Maple Syrup
1 /2 teaspoon	Ground Cinnamon
1 tablespoon	Vanilla Extract
1	Egg, beaten
2 tablespoons	Olive Oil/ Coconut Oil

Directions:

1. Combine mashed bananas and beaten egg in a bowl and mix until well incorporated.
2. Stir in honey/maple syrup, vanilla extract and cinnamon.
3. In a non-stick frying pan, heat oil over medium temperature.
4. Scoop pancake mixture using spoon and shape as pancake in the pan.
5. Cook each side for 2 to 3 minutes or until brown.
6. Top with your favorite fruit and drizzle with honey or maple syrup.

Coco Blueberry Oatmeal

Ingredients:

1 ½ cups	Shredded Coconut Meat
2	Ripe Bananas, peeled and cut into cubes
1 cup	Coconut Milk (Full Fat)
¼ cup	Coconut Butter
1 cup	Fresh or Frozen Blueberries
1 tablespoon	Gelatin

Directions:

1. Heat a medium pot in the stove.
2. Melt coconut butter and pour in coconut milk. Add vanilla and banana cubes. Season with salt. Mix until boiling.
3. Lower heat and simmer. Keep mixing until banana cubes are broken down into pieces.
4. Gradually add gelatin while mixing. Keep mixing until gelatin is properly dissolved.
5. Mix in blueberries and simmer for about 2 minutes.
6. Turn off heat but leave pot in the stove. Add shredded coconut meat.
7. Leave in the stove for 5 more minutes to soften coconut meat.
8. It can stay fresh in the refrigerator for up to 3 days.

Turkey Meatballs

Ingredients:

1lb	Ground Turkey
1 large	White Onion, minced
5 cloves	Garlic, minced
½ teaspoon	Dried Thyme
½ teaspoon	Dried Rosemary
1 handful	Fresh Basil
2 tablespoons	Soy Sauce
½ teaspoon	Salt
1 cup	Coconut Oil

Directions:

1. Mix all ingredients in a large bowl. Scoop with spoon and shape like a ball.
2. Heat coconut oil in a deep pot over medium temperature. Deep fry meatballs until golden brown.
3. You can use these meatballs to top your pasta dishes.
4. You can also serve it with soup if you desire.

Chapter 5 – Paleo Soup

Soups are easy to prepare and they are filling. They are versatile; you can turn almost anything into soup. During winter, having soup keeps you warm and comfortable. Soup dishes also help relieve colds and flu symptoms. These Paleo soup dishes are tasty and hearty; you can have them anytime of the day.

Mussels Soup

Ingredients:

2lbs	Fresh Mussels
1 inch	Ginger, crushed
5 cloves	Garlic, crushed
2 medium	White Onions, chopped
1 bunch	Lemongrass
½ teaspoon	Salt
2 tablespoons	Fish Sauce
3 tablespoons	Butter or Ghee
2 cups	Water

Directions:

1. In a deep pot, heat butter or ghee and sauté garlic, onions and ginger.
2. Add water. Increase heat, cover and boil.
3. Add lemongrass in boiling water for 5 to 10 minutes or until aromatic.
4. Remove lemongrass. Add mussels.
5. Season with salt and fish sauce.
6. Let boil until mussels are fully cooked.
7. Serve while hot.

Butternut Squash Soup

Ingredients:

2	Butternut Squash, gutted and halved
1 can	Coconut Milk
4 cups	Water
2 tablespoons	Coconut Oil
1 handful	Fresh Cilantro, chopped
1 tablespoon	Fresh Ginger, ground
2 teaspoons	Black Pepper, ground
2 teaspoons	Salt

Directions:

1. Brush the butternut squash meat with coconut oil. Roast in the oven at 350°F until tender.
2. Cool and spoon out flesh. Place in a Dutch oven or a large pot.
3. Add coconut milk and water. Puree with hand mixer or blend in batches.
4. Heat in the stove and simmer.
5. Add pepper, salt, ginger and cilantro. Reduce heat to low.
6. Mix thoroughly until all lumps are gone.
7. Top with cheese or toasted bacon bits.

Onion Soup

Ingredients:

4 large	White Onions
4 cups	Chicken Stock
½ cup	Coconut Milk
½ tablespoons	Balsamic Vinegar
1 tablespoon	Honey
2 tablespoons	Butter/Ghee
1 pinch	Black Pepper, ground
1 pinch	Salt

Directions:

1. Skin the onions and chop.
2. In a deep pot, melt butter or ghee over medium heat.
3. Sauté onions until wilted.
4. Add vinegar and honey. Mix vigorously.
5. Stir in chicken stock. Mix, cover and boil. Lower down heat.
6. Remove from heat and puree using a hand-held blender or immersion blender.
7. Bring back to stove and simmer in low heat.
8. Add coconut milk. Mix slowly and season with salt and pepper.
9. Best served when hot. You can pair it with your favorite roast dishes.

Carrot Zucchini Soup with Ginger

Ingredients:

4 cups	Vegetable Stock or Chicken Stock
1 cup	Coconut Milk
8	Carrots, peeled and chopped
2	Zucchinis, peeled and chopped
2 tablespoons	Ginger, minced
1	Red Onion, diced
1	Red Apple, peeled, seeded and chopped
1 teaspoon	Turmeric Powder
1 pinch	Cinnamon Powder
2 tablespoons	Butter, Lard or Ghee

Directions:

1. In a saucepan, melt butter, lard or ghee over medium heat.
2. Sauté ginger and onion for 2 minutes or until ginger is aromatic.
3. Stir in carrots, zucchini and apples. Mix thoroughly.
4. Season with cinnamon powder and turmeric powder.
5. Mix until carrots and zucchini are soft.
6. Pour in vegetable stock or chicken stock. Mix, cover and boil.
7. Lower heat and simmer. Remove from heat.
8. Puree until smooth using immersion blender or hand-held blender.
9. Pour coconut milk gradually and mix. Return to heat and simmer on low.
10. Serve hot or warm.

Mushroom Soup

Ingredients:

1 ½ lbs	Wild Mushrooms, sliced
7 cups	Chicken Stock
1 cup	Coconut Milk
2 large	Shallots, diced
¼ cup	Fresh Parsley, chopped
1 tablespoon	Fresh Thyme, chopped
2 tablespoons	Tapioca Starch
1 pinch	Black Pepper, ground
3 tablespoons	Ghee

Directions:

1. In a saucepan, heat ghee over medium temperature. Sauté shallots until soft.
2. Add mushrooms and thyme. Cook until mushrooms are moist.
3. Pour chicken stock and boil. Lower heat and simmer.
4. Gradually pour in coconut milk while stirring slowly. Season with salt and pepper.
5. Sprinkle with tapioca starch while mixing slowly to thicken the soup.
6. Turn off heat.
7. Serve with chopped parsley on top.

Chapter 6 – Paleo Salads

Fruits salads are refreshing and they are full of vitamins and nutrients that help your body function optimally. Fruits are also full of fiber that promotes better digestion. Better digestion means your body is able to absorb nutrients from the food that you eat and excrete unwanted toxins and residues. This leads to more effective weight loss and also prevents diseases and conditions related to digestion.

Citrus Fruit Salad

Ingredients:

6	Mandarin Oranges, peeled and segmented
4	Red Apples, seeded and diced
4	Kiwi, peeled and diced
½ cup	Blueberries, washed and drained
½ cup	Pomegranate Seeds
4 tablespoons	Lemon Juice, freshly squeezed
2 teaspoons	Poppy Seeds
½ cup	Avocado Oil

Directions:

1. In a mixing bowl, combine avocado oil, lemon juice and poppy seeds. Whisk until emulsified. Set aside.
2. In a large bowl, mix together all the fruits and drizzle with the dressing. Toss until all fruits are evenly coated.
3. Cool in the refrigerator for 30 minutes to an hour and serve.

Strawberry Broccoli Salad

Ingredients:

2 cups	Fresh Strawberries, halved
4 cups	Broccoli Florets, stemmed
¼ cup	Almonds, sliced
½ cup	Homemade Mayonnaise or Low-fat Mayonnaise
2	Red Onions, julienned
2 tablespoons	Lemon Juice, freshly squeezed
1 tablespoon	Poppy Seeds
1 tablespoon	Honey

Directions:

1. Mix honey, poppy seeds, lemon juice and mayonnaise in a bowl.
2. In a separate bowl, combine broccoli florets, strawberries, almonds and onions.
3. Drizzle dressing all over salad and mix until all are evenly coated.
4. Refrigerate for 30 minutes or more and serve cold.

Crunchy Grape and Apple Salad

Ingredients:

2	Pears, cored and diced
4	Red Apples, cored and diced
2 cups	Green Seedless Grapes, halved
¼ cup	Pine Nuts
1 stalk	Celery, diced
½ fruit	Lemon, juiced
½ teaspoon	Cinnamon
2 tablespoons	Olive Oil

Directions:

1. Combine pears, apples, grapes, nuts and celery in a deep bowl.

2. In a separate bowl, whisk together lemon juice, olive oil and celery until well blended.

3. Pour dressing all over salad and mix thoroughly.

4. Cool in the refrigerator for 30 minute or more and serve cold.

Strawberry Cucumber Salad

Ingredients:

4 cups	Fresh Strawberries, sliced thinly
2 large	Cucumbers, sliced into thin rounds
1 cup	Olive Oil
¼ cup	Apple Cider Vinegar
¼ cup	Honey
1 medium	White Onion, minced
1 teaspoon	Ground Dry Mustard
1 tablespoon	Poppy Seeds

Directions:

1. In a deep mixing bowl, whisk together olive oil, apple cider vinegar, honey, mustard, poppy seeds and onions.

2. In a separate bowl, mix together strawberries and cucumbers.

3. Gradually pour dressing while mixing to evenly coat everything.

4. Serve in individual salad plates.

Cranberry Greens Salad

Ingredients:

12 oz	Baby Spinach mixed with Arugula
2 large	Avocados, peeled, pitted and sliced
¾ cup	Roasted Almonds
¾ cup	Dried Cranberries
2/3 cup	Olive Oil
1 tablespoon	Poppy Seeds
½ teaspoon	Paprika
2 teaspoons	Dried Mustard
1 medium	Sweet Onion, minced
¼ cup	White Balsamic Vinegar
¼ cup	Honey
1 pinch	Salt
1 pinch	Ground Black Pepper

Directions:

1. In a deep bowl, mix olive oil, poppy seeds, paprika, dried mustard, sweet onion, white balsamic vinegar, honey, salt and pepper. Set aside.
2. In a salad bowl, place washed baby spinach and arugula. Mix in roasted almonds and dried cranberries.
3. Gradually pour in dressing while mixing to coat everything evenly.
4. Top with remaining roasted almonds and dried cranberries. Serve.

Chapter 7 – Paleo Lunches

Contrary to what you expect, Paleo lunches are not bland or boring. They are actually tasty, fun and enjoyable. These Paleo lunch recipes are easy to prepare, tasty, and healthy.

Orange N' Lemon Chicken

Ingredients:

4	Chicken Breasts, boneless and skinless
2 tablespoons	Lemon Juice, freshly squeezed
1 cup	Orange Juice, freshly squeezed
½ teaspoon	Salt
½ teaspoon	Ground Black Pepper
1 handful	Fresh Chives, chopped
4 sprigs	Fresh Thyme, chopped
2 cloves	Garlic, minced
1 tablespoon	Olive Oil

Directions:

1. In a deep bowl, mix together lemon juice, orange juice, pepper, salt and thyme.
2. Mix in chicken breasts and make sure they are all evenly coated. Marinate in the refrigerator for 4 to 8 hours or overnight.
3. Drain chicken and pat dry with paper towel.
4. Brush grill pan with olive oil and heat over medium temperature.
5. Cook chicken until golden brown on all sides.
6. Cut into thin slices and top with chives.
7. Serve while hot.

Seafood Zucchini Noodles

Ingredients:

4 medium	Zucchini noodles (use spiralizer)
1lb	Shrimps, precooked and tails removed
2 tablespoons	Coconut Oil
6 cups	Grape Tomatoes, cut into half
6 cloves	Garlic, minced
1 sprig	Fresh Basil, chopped
1 pinch	Salt
1 pinch	Ground Pepper

Directions:

1. In a large skillet, add coconut oil and heat over medium temperature.
2. Sauté garlic until it releases its aroma.
3. Turn heat to low. Add tomatoes and cook until soft.
4. Mix in precooked shrimps and simmer.
5. Add zucchini noodles, basil, pepper and salt. Mix until zucchini is soft.
6. Top with fresh basil.
7. Best served while hot.

Chicken Tomato with Basil

Ingredients:

4 thinly	Chicken Breasts, deboned, skinned and sliced
2 tablespoons	Ghee or Butter
2 cloves	Garlic, minced
4 large	Basil Leaves, chopped
1 cup	Cherry Tomatoes, cut in half

Directions:

1. Heat pan over medium temperature. Add ghee or butter and sauté cherry tomatoes until soft and wilted.
2. Add chicken slices. Mix thoroughly to make sure everything is coated with the tomato mixture.
3. Season with salt and pepper. Mix from time to time until chicken slices are thoroughly cooked.
4. Mix in garlic and basil.
5. Cook for 1 more minute and remove from heat.
6. Season with chopped basil and serve.

Slow Cooker Pot Roast

Ingredients:

3 lb	Chuck Roast
1 cup	Beef Stock
3 small	Carrots, chopped
3 cloves	Garlic, minced
1 large	Red Onion, sliced
2 tablespoons	Ghee or Butter
2 stalks	Celery, chopped
2 teaspoons	Cumin
1 teaspoon	Dried Oregano
½ teaspoon	Paprika
1 pinch	Ground Black Pepper
1 pinch	Salt

Directions:

1. Evenly coat chuck roast with paprika, cumin, salt, oregano and pepper.
2. In a pan, heat ghee or butter and sauté onions over medium heat.
3. Mix in garlic and sauté until fragrant. Toss in celery and carrots and cook until tender.
4. Place everything in the slow cooker.
5. Add beef stock, salt and pepper and set to low for 6 to 8 hours.

Roasted Salmon with Vinaigrette Dressing

Ingredients:

1 lb	Fresh Salmon
2 tablespoons	Avocado Oil
2 teaspoons	Lemon Juice, freshly squeezed
3 teaspoons	Walnut Oil
¼ teaspoon	Mustard
1 teaspoon	Ground Black Pepper
1 teaspoon	Salt
1 teaspoon	Dried Rosemary
1 teaspoon	Onion leeks, chopped

Directions:

1. Massage the salmon with salt, pepper and rosemary.
2. In a non-stick grill pan, heat avocado oil over medium temperature and cook each side of the salmon until golden brown. Set aside.
3. In a mixing bowl, whisk together walnut oil, lemon juice, mustard, salt and pepper.
4. Drizzle cooked salmon with vinaigrette dressing and top with onion leeks.

Chapter 8 – Paleo Snacks

There are no hard restrictions with Paleo snacks. In fact, you can just grab some fruits, mixed nuts or dried fruits. Enjoy your snack time with these irresistible Paleo snacks.

Roasted Cauliflower

Ingredients:

1 head	Cauliflower, stemmed and core removed
4 tablespoons	Olive Oil
1 teaspoon	Salt

Directions:

1. Preheat your oven to 425°F.
2. In a bowl, mix together salt and olive oil and mix in cauliflower florets until they are evenly coated.
3. Line your baking sheet with parchment paper and spread the cauliflower florets evenly. If you don't have time to prepare the cauliflowers, you can buy packed pre-cut cauliflower in the groceries.
4. Roast for an hour. Turn the florets about 3 to 4 times until golden brown.
5. If you want it sweeter, brown the florets more for better caramel taste.
6. Serve while hot.

Strawberry Ice Cream

Ingredients:

1 lb	Fresh Strawberries, cut into pieces
14 fl oz	Coconut Milk
1 tablespoon	Liquid Stevia to taste
½ tablespoon	Lemon Juice, freshly squeezed

Directions:

1. Process all ingredients in your blender or food processor until no strawberry pieces are present. Mixture should be smooth and creamy.
2. Transfer in old ice cream containers or any deep containers you have.
3. Freeze overnight. Since it has no sugar, it will be rock hard so thaw it in the refrigerator or room temperature for at least an hour before serving.

Eggs Guacamole

Ingredients:

4 large	Eggs, hard boiled
1 medium	Avocado, mashed
1 teaspoon	Lemon Juice
2 teaspoons	Hot Pepper Sauce
¼ teaspoon	Ground Black Pepper
¼ teaspoon	Salt

Directions:

1. Peel the hard boiled eggs and cut in the middle, lengthwise. Separate yolk using spoon and transfer in a bowl.
2. Mash the egg yolks and add the mashed avocados. Stir in hot sauce, lemon juice, salt and pepper.
3. Spoon out mixture and refill egg white.

Pizza Bites

Ingredients:

20 to 30 pieces	Large Pepperoni
1 cup	Pizza Sauce
1 cup	Grated Cheese
¼ cup	Black Olives
1 large	Bell Pepper, chopped
½ cup	Mushrooms, sliced thinly
¼ cup	Green Onions, minced

Directions:

1. Set your oven to 400°F.
2. Arrange the pepperoni slices in your baking sheet and roast for 8 minutes on both sides, turning over once.
3. While the pepperoni is roasting in the oven, prepare the rest of the ingredients.
4. When done, arrange toppings on top of the pepperoni slices.
5. Bring back to the oven and bake for 5 to 10 minutes or until cheese has melted.
6. You can store your leftovers in a container and freeze them. Just reheat when needed.

Avocado Crunchies

Ingredients:

1 medium	Avocado, halved and pitted
1 handful	Sunflower Seeds, coat removed
1 pinch	Salt
1 teaspoon	Avocado Oil

Directions:

1. In a non-stick pan, roast sunflower seeds for 5 minutes or until brown. Season with salt.
2. Add avocado oil and mix until all are evenly coated.
3. Roast until golden brown.
4. Set aside and cool.
5. Refill the avocado halves with roasted sesame seeds. Serve.

Chapter 9 – Paleo Dinners

Dinner must be fulfilling, satisfying, and nutritious to help you get started the next day. These Paleo dinner recipes are not only nutritious and filling, but they are also easy to prepare and super tasty.

Comfort Soup for the Soul

Ingredients:

2 lbs	Sweet Potatoes, peeled and chopped
4 slices	Bacon, cooked and diced
½ cup	Coconut Milk
2 cups	Chicken Stock
1 teaspoon	Ginger, ground
1 tablespoon	Ground Cinnamon
1 tablespoon	Nutmeg, ground

Directions:

1.   In a slow cooker, add chicken stock, sweet potatoes, nutmeg, ginger and cinnamon. Mix well and set to low. Cook for 6 hours.

2.   When cooked, add coconut milk and blend using a hand-held mixer or immersion blender until creamy.

3.   Top with bacon bits and serve.

Pulled Pork with Coleslaw

Ingredients:

For Barbecue Sauce

24oz	Canned Tomatoes, drained
6oz	Tomato Paste
2 tablespoons	Ghee
¼ cup	Honey
1/3 cup	Apple Cider Vinegar
1/3 cup	Blackstrap Molasses
2 tablespoons	Ground Mustard
2 tablespoons	Chili Powder
1 tablespoon	Garlic Powder
1 tablespoon	Onion Powder
1 teaspoon	Salt

For Pulled Pork

4 lbs	Pork Shoulder, excess fat removed
1	Yellow Onion, sliced thinly
1 pinch	Salt

For Coleslaw

1 pack	Pre-packed Coleslaw Vegetables
¼ cup	Honey
½ cup	Apple Cider Vinegar
1/3 cup	Olive Oil
¼ teaspoon	Garlic Powder
½ teaspoon	Celery Seeds
1 teaspoon	Salt

Directions:

1.   Melt ghee in a pot over medium heat. Add all ingredients for the Barbecue sauce and simmer. Mix from time to time to avoid burning. Set aside.

2.   In a slow cooker, place pork shoulder and pour barbecue sauce. Add onions and salt. Mix until entire pork is covered with sauce. Set on low and cook for 8 hours. When cooked, use fork to shred meat off of the bone. Place in a serving plate and set aside.

3.   In a large, deep bowl, mix together honey, olive oil, apple cider vinegar, celery seeds, garlic powder and salt. Add coleslaw vegetables and toss to coat everything.

4.   Serve with coleslaw on the side.

Crunchy Coconut Chicken Salad

Ingredients:

2 large	Chicken Breast Fillets
2 tablespoons	Coconut Flour
2 tablespoons	Coconut Flakes, unsweetened
1 large	Egg, beaten
2 cups	Mixed Salad Greens
1 teaspoon	Honey
1 pinch	Salt
1 pinch	Ground Black Pepper
2 tablespoon	Coconut Oil
3 tablespoons	Olive Oil
3 tablespoons	Apple Cider Vinegar

Directions:

1.   Prepare 3 bowls to use for breading/dredging. Place coconut flour in the first bowl, beaten egg on the second bowl and coconut flakes on the third.

2.   Heat coconut oil in a skillet over medium heat.

3.   Dredge chicken fillet in coconut flour then on the beaten egg. Make sure fillet is evenly coated. Lastly, dredge in coconut flakes and make sure everything is well coated.

4.   Cook fillet in hot skillet until golden brown and cooked through and through.

5.   In a mixing bowl, combine honey and apple cider vinegar. Add olive oil gradually while whisking. Keep whisking until mixture is creamy. Add salt and pepper.

6.   Place mixed salad greens in a mixing bowl and drizzle with ½ of the dressing. Toss to cover everything.

7.   Transfer in a serving bowl and place chicken on top. Serve with dressing on the side.

8.   Season with salt and pepper.

Cabbage Rolls

Ingredients:

½ lb	Ground Pork
10	Cabbage Leaves
1 clove	Garlic, minced
½ large	Onion, minced
1 tablespoon	Almond Meal
1	Egg, beaten
2 tablespoons	Coconut Aminos
2 tablespoons	Rice Vinegar
1 to 2 cups	Chicken Broth

Directions:

1.   In a large bowl, arrange cabbage leaves. Pour boiling water into the bowl. Make sure all the cabbage leaves are covered. Leave for 5 minutes until leaves are wilted. Remove leaves from water and set aside.

2.   In a deep mixing bowl, add pork, garlic, onion, vinegar, egg, coconut aminos and almond meal. Use your hands to mix all the ingredients together.

3.   Form 10 meatballs and set aside.

4.   Place one meatball in the middle of one cabbage leaf. Fold each side of the leaf to cover the meatball and tuck underneath. Do the same with the rest of the meatballs and cabbage leaves.

5.   In a stock pot, arrange the cabbage rolls. Add enough chicken broth to cover the cabbage rolls. Cover and set stove to medium heat.

6.   Cook for 20 to 25 minutes or until meatballs are cooked through and through.

7.   Serve while hot.

Roasted Chicken in Lemon and Thyme

Ingredients:

2 large	Chicken Breasts, skin and bones removed
1	Lemon
7 sprigs	Fresh Thyme, stems removed
1 tablespoon	Olive Oil
1 pinch	Salt
1 pinch	Ground Black Pepper

Directions:

1.   Place chicken in a ziplock bag or sealable container. Squeeze lemon over chicken.

2.   Add olive oil, thyme, salt and pepper. Zip container and shake vigorously to coat chicken evenly. Marinate in the refrigerator for 30 minutes to 8 hours.

3.   Preheat your oven to 350°F.

4.   Drizzle baking dish with olive oil. Place chicken in the baking dish and drizzle with more olive oil.

5.   Bake for 30 minutes or until chicken is brown on the sides.

6.   Place on serving plate and season with pepper and salt.

Beef Stew

Ingredients:

1.5 lbs	Lean Beef Meat, cut into large cubes
1 cup	Onion, sliced
3 tablespoons	Garlic, minced
2 tablespoons	Grass-fed Butter
1 tablespoon	Coconut Oil
1 tablespoon	Balsamic Vinegar
2 tablespoons	Arrowroot Powder
1 teaspoon	Garlic Powder
1 pinch	Salt
1 pinch	Ground Black Pepper
1 small	Sweet Potato, cut into chunks
8oz	Mushrooms, sliced
2 stems	Celery, diced
1 leaf	Bay Leaf
4 cups	Beef Broth

Directions:

1.   In a large, deep pot or Dutch oven, melt coconut oil over medium heat and sauté garlic and onion.

2.   In a bowl, place beef meat and season with salt and pepper. Mix to combine.

3.   Meanwhile, heat a skillet and melt 1 tablespoon butter. Sear beef meat on each side until brown. Remove from heat and add into the Dutch oven.

4.   Add 3 cups beef broth and adjust heat to low.

5.   Add sweet potato, bay leaf and celery. Mix to combine.

6.   Using the same skillet you used for searing, melt remaining butter and mix in the mushrooms. Adjust heat to medium and cook until soft.

7.   While cooking mushrooms, place 2 tablespoons arrowroot powder in Mason jar and fill with remaining beef broth. Cover lid and shake hard to dissolve powder.

8.   Add balsamic vinegar into the pan with mushroom and mix to coat everything.

9.   Add arrowroot mixture into the pan and mix until it turns into thick gravy.

10.   When done, transfer into the Dutch oven. Set stove to low and simmer for two hours or until meat is tender. Mix from time to time to prevent burning.

11.   Best served while hot.

Baked Pork Loin with Apples

Ingredients:

3	Thick Boneless Pork Loins
1 cup	Onions, diced
1 tablespoon	Garlic, minced
2 small	Green Apples, sliced
1 teaspoon	Italian Seasoning
1 pinch	Salt
1 pinch	Ground Pepper
1 tablespoon	Coconut Oil
½ cup	Pork Broth

Directions:

1. In a saucepan, heat ½ of the coconut oil over medium heat. Add pork loins and brown on each side. Set aside on a plate.

2. In the same saucepan, melt remaining coconut oil and sauté garlic and onions.

3. Add apple slices and season with salt, pepper and Italian seasonings. Set aside.

4. Preheat your oven to 350°F.

5. Arrange pork loins in the baking dish. Top with apple mixture. Add pork broth and cook for 30 minutes or until pork is tender.

Chapter 10 – Paleo Desserts

If you think Paleo is boring, think again. You can still have you favorite desserts but healthier and easy to prepare. These dessert recipes will make you wonder if you are really on a diet.

Chocolate Brownie Bites

Ingredients:

1/3 cup	Cocoa Powder, unsweetened
1 cup	Pitted Dates
1 ½ cups	Walnuts
1 teaspoon	Vanilla
1 pinch	Salt

Directions:

1. In a food processor or blender, process the walnuts and salt until finely ground.
2. Add cocoa powder, vanilla and dates. Process until everything is well combined.
3. While the blender or food processor is working, add water gradually to thicken the mixture and make them stick together. Do not put too much.
4. Transfer the mixture in a bowl. Scrape off remaining mixture using spatula.
5. Scoop out some mixture using spoon and form into balls using your hands.
6. You can store them in an airtight container and keep in the refrigerator for a week.

Banana Muffin with Sticky Date Ganache

Ingredients:

2 tablespoons	Butter/Ghee for greasing the muffin tray
2 medium	Ripe Bananas, peeled and chopped
3 tablespoons	Coconut Flour
12	Dates
1 tablespoon	Vanilla Extract
1 teaspoon	Honey
½ teaspoon	Baking Powder
2 medium	Eggs
10 tablespoons	Water

Sticky Date Ganache

6	Dates, chopped
½ fruit	Orange, juiced
3 tablespoons	Coconut Milk or Almond Milk
1 teaspoon	Vanilla Extract
1 teaspoon	Honey
	Raspberries, for garnish

Directions:

1. Preheat oven to 365°F.
2. Grease muffin tin with butter or ghee.
3. In a saucepan, simmer water and dates over low heat. When the dates have broken down and start to thicken, mash them with fork and set aside.
4. In a food processor or blender, process coconut flour, banana, egg, vanilla extract and baking powder. Mix until aerated and well combined.

5. Mix the date mixture to the banana mixture.
6. Transfer into the muffin tins and cook for 20 to 25 minutes or until brown on the sides.
7. While cooking the muffin, heat the sticky date ganache ingredients in a small bowl over medium temperature until the dates break down. Mash the dates with fork and whisk until thick.
8. Let the muffins cool for 5 minutes or until warm to touch before scooping a dollop of sticky date ganache on top of them. Garnish with raspberries.
9. You can store the muffins and toppings separately in airtight containers and use when needed. It can stay fresh up to 1 week in the refrigerator.

Triple Delight Truffle

Ingredients:

3 tablespoons	Pure Cocoa Powder, unsweetened
1 tablespoon	Ground Coffee
½ cup	Coconut Butter
1 tablespoon	Coconut Flakes, unsweetened
1 teaspoon	Honey
1 tablespoon	Coconut Oil

Directions:

1. Melt coconut butter in low temperature on the stove. Set aside
2. In a deep bowl, mix together cocoa powder, ground coffee, coconut flakes, honey and coconut butter. Mix thoroughly using fork or whisker.
3. Grease the ice cube tray with coconut oil and spoon some of the mixture in each hole. Pat the mixture flat using fork.
4. Freeze for 4 to 5 hours or overnight.
5. Defrost for 15 to 20 minutes in the refrigerator or room temperature before serving.
6. You can store it up to a month in the freezer as long as it is kept in an air-tight container.

Sunbutter Truffles

Ingredients:

5 tablespoons	Sunflower Seed Butter or Sunbutter
¾ cup	Almond Flour
1 tablespoon	Flaxseed Meal
½ cup	Chocolate Chips
1 tablespoon	Cacao Butter
1 tablespoon	Coconut Oil
1 tablespoon	Raw Honey
2 teaspoons	Vanilla Extract
1 pinch	Salt
¼ cup	Chopped Almonds

Directions:

1. In a large bowl, mix together sunflower seed butter, honey, vanilla, coconut oil, flaxseed meal, almond flour and salt. If you see oil rising on top of the butter, that's natural. Just mix the oil and butter together before adding it into the bowl. Mix thoroughly until well incorporated.
2. Scoop out dough and roll into balls. Line them in a baking pan with parchment paper and cool in the refrigerator for 30 minutes.
3. Meanwhile, melt chocolate chips over low heat and add cacao butter.
4. Dip each truffle in the melted chocolate and put back in the baking pan.
5. Sprinkle with chopped almonds and refrigerate until firm.
6. It will last longer if kept frozen in a sealed container. Defrost for a few minutes before serving.

Chocolate Almond Delight

Ingredients:

¼ cup	Unsweetened Shredded Coconut, more for garnish
1 cup	Raw Almonds
1 cup	Toasted Hazelnuts
1 ½ cups	Dates, pitted and chopped
2/3 cup	Raw Almond Butter
½ teaspoon	Vanilla Extract
5 tablespoons	Unsweetened Cocoa Powder

Directions:

1. In a food processor or blender, blend almonds, hazelnuts, dates, almond butter, vanilla extract and cocoa powder.
2. Blend until smooth. Scrape down the sides from time to time.
3. Transfer in a bowl and add shredded coconut. Mix until well incorporated.
4. Line your mini muffin tin with plastic wrap. Scoop out mixture with spoon and form into mounds.
5. Freeze for 3 to 5 hours or overnight.
6. Sprinkle with shredded coconut.
7. This dessert can stay fresh for more than 2 weeks when kept frozen in a tightly sealed container.

Conclusion

Paleo Diet has gotten a lot of attention lately due to its health benefits. For some, knowing that this diet can help them reduce weight and control their symptoms is enough reason to follow. But Paleo is more than that. It requires you to change your lifestyle and be more aware of your choices. With Paleo, you go back to eating what is good for your body and reverse the effects of a junk **diet** to start living a healthier lifestyle.

As saw by the recipes found in this cookbook, Paleo diet lets you enjoy the usual foods that you eat but in a healthier way. The food that you eat affects your overall health. When you eat clean foods, your body absorbs nutrients that it needs to function properly.

You do not have to go broke when you go Paleo. You can always substitute your ingredients with what is in season and more affordable. The ingredients for the recipes in this cookbook are easy to find and can be easily substituted.

If you enjoyed this book, please don't forget to share your thoughts with your friends, colleagues, and me by posting a review on Amazon. It will be greatly appreciated.

Thank you for buying this book!

Best wishes,

Erin Bloomfield

www.ingramcontent.com/pod-product-compliance
Lightning Source LLC
Chambersburg PA
CBHW050759240726
48654CB00008B/552